Rapid Weight Loss Affirmations

Positive Affirmations to Build a better Realationship With Food, Lose weight Fast, Stop Emotional Eating, Control Food Cravings and Solve your Sugar Addiction

Women's Meditation and Self-Care Institute

1

COPYRIGHT

Contents

A better relationship with Food

Every person and every culture has a particular relationship with food. Every living thing values food, but its most important to us humans.

Food has social effects, and there are different rituals about its consumption. No matter who you are or where you come from, or the kind of environment you grew in, food remains an integral part of life. Across the world, the ceremony of food is performed up to 3 times a day, including breakfast, lunch, and dinner.

Most people minimize their value for food by saying, "I don't like food. I only eat to live; I wish there were pills I could take to keep life going." However, sentiments like these are very exceptional. For many people, food creates different associations and meanings, some of which are formed when we are very young to notice.

Consider a toddler sitting on the table and refusing to eat his food. What will the mum say?

"Eat all your food; that's a good boy." "But I am full, mummy."

"Eat all your food to show mummy how much you love her..."

Most of us have been here, right? Being here as a parent is very tough. Especially when our children reach a certain age where they start creating boundaries. Well, this concern of food creates an association in our minds. We equalize food with love. We believe that food is the way we can show that someone is truly loved.

In many cultures, food is the center of every celebration. Weddings, engagements, birthdays, anniversaries, and even bar mitzvahs. Almost every special occasion worship food.

In certain cultures, food plays a social and ceremonial role, particularly in African communities. To understand your relationship with food, you should understand the type of culture you grew up in or what you are currently part of. To understand, ask yourself the following questions:

- What did my parents tell us about food when I was young?

- How did we celebrate with food? Did we use to eat together or celebrate with food?

- Has food been my fallback whenever bad things happen to me?

- Discovering your Relationship with Food
-

Discovering how you associate with food is a complex category that would take a single session to tackle or take several sessions to fully recover. The idea of this process is to simply discover what your relationship with overeating and emotions is.

The underlying truth is that many of us use food to overcome challenges in life. When having a lot of stress, we tend to find solace in sugar. This is because stress always burns glucose reserves, thus, creating a deficit in the body. The glucose reserves are the emergency supplies of the body. This means that one we are done with them, the body gets super hungry, telling us to look for more sugar.

When you get too stressed, you tend to burn glucose faster than usual. This leaves you constantly hungry. Thus, you end up craving for snacks like candy bars to replace the used glucose.

Another perspective explains why we depend on food when stressed, you see, the body always tends to balance the moods or negative energy with serotonin, a body hormone commonly referred to as the "happy hormone." While this seems good, the hormone creates intense cravings for sugar, which is responsible for increasing the serotonin amount in the body.

Therefore, it is important to consume healthy foods that produce serotonin, including spinach, tuna, celery, and poultry. Other important foods are fermented drinks and foods, and protein.

But there is also an issue with the stress that is beyond what we consume. When you are stressed, you release three hormones: norepinephrine, adrenaline, and cortisol. When you become stressed about a certain danger, these hormones are responsible for the flight and fight response. Because of such danger, the body holds onto any available fat just in case you need it for emergency response, i.e., in case you run out of food. Although this mechanism is great, it may cause weight gain in the case of long-term stress.

Apart from stress, there are other emotional eating components. The majority of us use food to overcome negative emotions.

For instance, consider the typical American stereotype of a woman who gets dumped by the boyfriend. The woman goes out with her girlfriends and takes drinks to forget her troubles. The rest of the time, she would get back home and eat a whole box of pizza, ice cream, and chocolate.

This stereotype has become ingrained in us culturally, thanks to social influence and modern advertising. This concept of food has been used by advertisers to sell their products

Another common situation that would result in weight gain is depression. There is an intimate link between depression and weight gain due to psychological and biochemical reasons.

When dealing with depression, or just feeling down, you may make bad food choices, which would create a negative spiral. Therefore, it is important to take care of one's emotional component to succeed in weight loss through hypnosis.

Healing Your Relationship with Food

Amidst the spiraling negative emotions when it comes to food, there is still hope to improve the existing relationship. The path to healing may be prolonged, but it takes your faith, your willingness, and dedicated yourself to hypnosis that will ensure you see the light at the end of the tunnel.

Several strategies can be implemented to improve your relationship with food, including:

Being Present

Many people practice unhealthy eating habits from their unconscious state of mind. It is very rare to binge on food when you are present at the moment.

When you stay present while eating, your body will signal you when you are full. It is also difficult to starve yourself if you are keen on your body's cues because the body will let you know when it is hungry. However, to listen to these cues, we must always be awake.

The cure for weight loss, which is promoted by hypnosis, is awareness. Poor eating habits mean that part of you check out. It is, therefore, time to check-in.

Learn to slow down your pace of eating food, as well as your pace in life. The more you become present with your meals, the more present you will be with your emotions and feelings that need attention. Often, these unattended emotions are the ones that drive our unwanted eating habits. Practice daily to be acquainted with being present. It may be difficult, but the rewards are excellent over some time.

Communication with Your Body

You must listen to your body the same way you would to an important person. If you fail to recognize your body's language, it is high time that you start getting curious. Learn the quirks and understand the non-verbal language. If, for instance, you get gassy once you eat pork, your body may be telling you that it has trouble digesting dairy products. If you ignore the message, the body may react even louder.

Just like couples always go for counseling to learn how to have effective communication, your body needs better communication. We can build trust with our bodies once we improve our communication with them. With hypnosis, our body can gain trust that we are listening to it and will naturally relax around food because of the less threat it feels.

Also, you need to ensure that you listen to your body's cues for affection, connection, and intimacy. Once you meet these needs, we will never associate them with hunger pangs.

Spend Quality Time with Food

You need an incredible amount of resources and energy to grow, harvest, prepare, and serve food to eat it. Considering this perspective, food deserves respect. Once in a while, spend time in the garden and understand what it takes for a particular food to grow from nature and get ready for harvest. Visit your nearest market and talk to the farmers about your favorite foods. Create a strong relationship with food and where they are grown.

Forgive Yourself and Food

Whatever the relationship you have had with food, forgive yourself and forgive food. Let your bad past be. You have done your best over time, and it is now time to start all over again. This does not mean that you will eat perfectly perfectly. It only means that you are enabling your life journey to be imperfect without blaming yourself for every mistake.

When you forgive yourself, you can start with a newer perspective. You will let go of the past judgments you made about yourself and food to develop some compassion. It is time to forgive yourself for the mistakes you have made with your body and food.

Don't fight with food and be kind and gentle with yourself. In case you hate food because it becomes your substitute whenever you are facing frustration, permit yourself to have comfort. Understand that you are an imperfect human being who has difficulties.

Rate Your Satiety Level on a Scale of 10

Every day, check with yourself where you are with being physically full, with one being famished and ten being full to the gills. Ideally, being below 2 or 3 is not recommended, as this can result in light-headedness and might affect your immune system. This level of fullness might also make you descend upon food in a manner that would lead to overeating. Also, reaching the level above 6 or 7 might also not be the best since it would result in discomfort and maybe a sign of emotional eating rather than for physical purposes.

Be Informed About Your Emotional Triggers to Food

If your satiety level is above 7, it is important to ask yourself, "what reason am I hungry? What was I thinking about? What am I feeling now?" These questions are very important because sometimes we feel hungry because we are bored, or lonely, or angry, or self-deprived, or anxious. You must address these needs instead of eating to cope with them.

Love Your Food

With hypnosis, you will understand that food is not the enemy. People who suffer from illicit drug or alcohol abuse are able to abstain from these substances completely. However, with food, it is difficult to have abstinence since eating is key to survival. Similar to our goals in relationships, we strive to have a healthy boundary with food, so that we are neither hedonistic or too rigid.

It might be illuminating to ask the following questions: How do I relate with food? Am I obsessive? Am I demanding? Am I avoidant? If your answers are yes, then you need to explore these issues further with hypnosis. Listen carefully to yourself and check the symptoms in order to look for a long-term strategy.

List down the Strategies That Can Heal You Without Emotional Eating

You may need a simple warm bath. Or maybe call a friend or get so sleep.

Address that investment problem you have been dodging. You can keep the long list on your locker or on your phone, where you can frequently refer to whenever you need it.

Choose the Words You Use Carefully

When you frequently use the words such as "I can't," "should," and "I have tossed," such as "I need to cut down on my food intake," or "I have to stop eating in order to lose weight," can pull you back. This is associated with the fact that your inner body will be fighting against your critical voice. The words above may be rewarded with more compelling statements like "I choose to not eat so much," or "I am starting to work out today." This means growth because you will be reframing your discomfort as growth and telling yourself that you can handle your weight loss journey amidst the discomfort.

Be Ready and Willing to Face Life Head-On

When you tend to indulge in eating every time you are faced with challenges, it means you are hiding out from life challenges. By developing a healthy relationship with food, you will not be able to use it as a form of distraction. Being attentive to your emotions, however unpleasant they might be, will help you avoid overeating while also addressing your problems.

Weight Loss Myths

Food and Weight Loss Myths that Will Stop You from Losing Weight When practicing hypnosis, we need to give our body the right food, even as we cut down on sugar and high-calorie foods. However, there are weight loss diet tips that many people perceive as healthy, yet they are in fact, myths that we should stop believing. Keeping off these myths will help you lose weight efficiently as well as ensure you remain healthy in the long run.

Myth #1 Skipping meals can help you lose weight

It is necessary that you eat proper meals throughout the day to have a good metabolism, which results in rapid weight loss. Skipping meals, particularly breakfast, is bad for you since you may overindulge later in the day, which may result in weight gain.

Myth #2 All calories are bad

All calories that are found in foods have similar energy content because a calorie is the measurement of energy. However, it does not mean that the sources of calories (the foods we eat) have similar effects on weight.

Different foods have different metabolic pathways, and as a result, can have different effects on the hormones regulating our body weights as well as hunger.

For instance, the calories that we obtain from proteins are different from those that we find from carbs or fats. Replacing fats and carbs with proteins will help boost your metabolism rate and reduce your craving, while also regulating the function of the hormones that control your weight.

Also, calories from fruits and vegetables tend to be many fillings compared to those obtained from manufactured foods like bread, cakes, and candy.

Myth #3 Carbs can make you fat

Having a low-carb diet can lead to rapid weight loss. In many instances, this always happens even without restricting oneself from the number of calories consumed. As long as the overall carb intake remains low while the protein intake remains high, you are able to lose weight.

This does not mean that carbs cause weight gain. Although cases of obesity started being reported around the 1980s, people have been eating carbs even before this era. In fact, carbs from whole foods are considered healthy. Furthermore, removing a full food group from your diet would

Myth #4 Stay away from fats in order to lose weight

Most people fear eating fats because they associate them with weight gain. Fat has about nine calories per gram compared to only four calories in proteins or carbs. Fat is usually common in junk foods and is very calorie-dense. Yet, when you take calorie within a healthy range, then it cannot cause weight gain.

Also, diets that have high-fat content have been proven to cause weight loss compared to those with high carb-content. Unhealthy fatty, junk foods, however, will definitely make you fat.

Myth #5 Breaking your meal into smaller portions can cause weight loss It is a common myth that taking meals in smaller, frequent portions can lead to weight loss. However, this is not the case because what matters the most is the total amount of calorie intake, whether it is taken in a single meal or in six meals.

Myth #6 Eating breakfast is key to weight loss

Many researchers have proven that those who skip breakfast are more likely to weight more compared to breakfast eaters. However, this is because those who take breakfast have the tendency to engage in healthier lifestyle habits. It is also a myth that taking breakfast can boost your metabolism. It is best to eat

17

only when you are hungry and stop whenever you feel full. You can always eat breakfast when you want to, but you should not expect that it can have a significant effect on your weight.

Solving your Sugar Addiction with Hypnosis

Many people are currently suffering from sugar addiction, and this largely contributes to the rising cases of overweight and obesity. Hypnosis will enable you to deal with sugar addiction in an effective and fast manner. Most sugar addiction habits develop during childhood as a way of eliminating calmness or discomfort.

When we are young, we love sugary foods because they make us feel better. And as we grow older, the same sweetness helps us get happy due to the released happy hormones. However, the more amounts of sugar we consume, the more we will need to release happy hormones.

The Negative Impacts of Sugar Addiction

Sugary foods are the major contributors to weight gain, particularly those that are not nutritious. They will increase the risks of diseases such as teeth rotting, heart diseases, and diabetes as you add weight. By breaking sugar eating habits, you will be able to lead a healthier life. Hypnosis can, thus, help you to:

- Feel less worried and calmer about the sugar effects such as for overweight or obesity

- Begin utilizing strategies that can control the type of food you consume

- Resist the urge to eat sweet things and make healthier choices

- Start admiring foods that have low levels of sugar

- Feel better because of regained metabolism rate

Solving Sugar Addiction with Hypnosis

You can easily treat sugar addiction with proper hypnosis. Through the guidance of experienced hypnotherapy, you will be able to let go of the bad habit. Taking sugar is usually a personal or individual choice, which you can only solve by yourself.

Hypnosis can help you establish the cause of your love or addiction for sugar. It will enable you to become conscious of the state of your mind and body every time you think of taking sugar. With positive suggestions, you will be able to consider alternative ways to cope with your cravings.

LOSE WEIGHT FAST AND NATURALLY

The idea of hypnosis is usually to turn off they crave for foods that are unhealthy, and instead adopting a healthy lifestyle. By utilizing hypnotherapy, one can get empowered to change the automatic thoughts that trigger unhealthy cravings. Overeating and overindulgence in food are always associated with certain emotional feelings, events, and relationships. The mind convinces us that when we're in some situations, food serves as the key objective. For instance, when stressed, food acts as consolation. To stay away from such habits, we must access these unconscious habits, remove them, and replace them with meaningful thoughts that prevent overeating or overindulgence. Thus, hypnosis empowers us to realize the negative thoughts and instead create positive associations that result in long term good results in weight reduction.

How the mind is Invaded with Food

Using Hypnosis to Overcome the Mental Barriers Jude had started a diet plan and was in a position to see results in weeks. When she saw the flat tummy of her and toned arms, she felt great.

But something changed. Jude got a new job, and all over sudden, she found it extremely challenging to lose even an inch. With time, she started to overindulge, stopped counting calories, and craved for food items that are unhealthy. Her wait began to stall, and she completely fell off the diet.

What could have happened to Jude? She started strong, but she couldn't stay on track for an extended time. If we assess her situation, we might identify a habit pattern, which explains her behavior.

We create habit patterns through repetition, and with time, they start to be automatic responses to the planet. Jude likely developed a pattern of emotional eating, which inhibited her from attaining the weight loss goals of her. Food became Jude's automatic response to work-related stress in the new working environment of her. These habits of the mind are precisely why it's quite challenging for a lot of us to lose weight.

Deep in the minds of ours, we've strong ideas that keep us thinking of unhealthy behaviors. With time, folks train the mind to think that unhealthy behaviors, as in the case of emotional eating or overindulging, are the necessary behaviors to maintain our well-being. And as such, if the mind repeatedly thinks of these behaviors, long term changes start to be difficult.

As in the case of Jude, emotional eating is simply an example of associations that negatively impact our attempts to lose weight. There are many other associations that individuals develop, which impact the relationship of theirs with food negatively. Several of these associations that hinder weight loss include:

- Food and constant eating helps in distracting us from anxiety, anger, and sadness

- Food is a comforting tool; it comforts us when we're feeling sad or perhaps stressed

- Overeating unhealthy or sugary foods are associated with times that are good and celebrations

- Unhealthy and sugary foods are a reward

- Overeating can help anyone to conquer the fear that you will not manage to lose weight

Food is a source of entertainment when you are feeling bored Ultimately, losing weight effectively with the use of hypnosis requires we assess these root causes, understand them, and finally reframe them. This Is just what hypnosis is able to do!

Reframing The Addiction of yours to Food using Hypnosis The first step of a hypnosis process is actually: To recognize the reason why you haven't been in a position to achieve the weight loss goals of yours. Just how does this happen? To be able to understand the shortfalls of yours, a hypnotherapist will generally ask you questions that are associated with the eating behaviors of yours and the weight loss journey of yours. This process of info gathering is going to help you determine what you may have to change to attain the goal of yours.

After understanding your eating habits, a hypnotherapist will guide you through an induction process, which entails the relaxation of the mind and body, in which you are going to enter a hypnotic state. While in the state, the mind of yours is going to become highly suggestible, you'll have shed of your conscious, critical mind, giving the hypnotherapist the chance to speak directly to the subconscious mind of yours.

In hypnosis, you'll be provided with positive affirmations and suggestions, and you might be asked to visualize changes. There are many good suggestions for fast weight loss, including:

Identify the possible unconscious eating habits - With hypnosis, you will be in a position to determine the negative unconscious eating patterns you've developed over time. When you're hypnotized, you can easily be more mindful of what makes you eat food that is unhealthy and then come up with strategies to help change the habit.

Reframing your inner voice - With hypnosis, you are going to be in a position to speak with the internal voice, which is actually misleading you to eat food that is bad. Not merely can a hypnotherapist help you speak with the inner voice, but he/she can also turn your inner voice right into a support system that guides you to consider rational and positive suggestions.

Developing healthy coping tactics - With hypnosis, you will be able to develop healthy ways to cope with stress. During hypnosis, you will become conscious of the fact that snacking isn't the only method of dealing with worry and anxiety. You'll, therefore, consider other coping strategies.

Improve the choices of yours of meals - You may be addicted to junk food, but with hypnosis, you are going to be in a position to get the low for healthier foods

Encouraging healthy eating - With hypnosis, you'll develop the practice of choosing healthier eating habits like reducing the food portion sizes of yours or perhaps rehearsing certain eating choices like taking the remaining food home when you're eating in a restaurant.

Visualizing success - A hypnotic program will encourage you to visualize exactly how you can achieve weight loss goals. When you visualize exactly how it feels to lose weight, you will have higher chances of practicing the weight-loss tactics.

Boost the confidence of yours - With hypnosis, you are going to be in a position to develop positive suggestions that boost your confidence. With confidence, you are going to be in a position to achieve the weight loss goals of yours.

Identifying the unconscious indicators - With a hypnotic therapy, you are going to be in a position to identify the signals you will get from the body of yours. It will help you figure out when you're full and be in a position to determine the difference between feeling hungry and thirsty.

When doing hypnosis, these recommendations can help you to conquer the cravings of yours and bad eating habits. Not all of them apply to every individual. The goal, nonetheless, is actually to develop a hypnosis plan, which includes the suggestions that are only relevant to you.

How Hypnosis helps you Achieve Rapid Weight Loss During hypnosis, your mind becomes open to any suggestions. Research indicates that when in the hypnotic state, your mind is more likely to experience exciting changes, which allows learning about the info you're receiving without having to think consciously or critically.

With this state, you're always detached from the conscious mind of yours, thus, you do not interrupt the thoughts of yours with the question about what you're hearing. And this's how hypnosis helps with the breaking down of barriers which prevent you from shedding off pounds.

In hypnotherapy, repetition is the key to success. This explains the reason many hypnotherapists provide you with self-hypnosis recordings, which you own to listen to repeatedly. The barriers in the brain are always very powerful, and only through repeated hypnosis can you untangle yourself from the convictions.

Hypnosis teaches the brain how to think differently about eating and food. The suggestions we discussed above can enable you to achieve the following:

Control Food Cravings

Weight loss hypnotic technique is able to help you to detach yourself from cravings and isolate yourself from food items that are unhealthy. For example, during hypnosis, you may be asked to visualize exactly how you are going to send away the cravings. Suggestions are able to help in reframing cravings and teach you how you can handle them in an effective way.

Success

Expectations of an individual dictate his/her reality. With the hope of success, we're apt to take the actions necessary to attain success. Hypnosis is able to plant this seed of success in the mind of yours, thus, providing you with the unconscious power to keep yourself on course.

Positivity

No one loves negativity, and our brains are actually no different. Negative thoughts are able to spoil your dedication and ability to lose weight. Through hypnosis, you are going to become conscious of the food items that you cannot eat. These food items don't help your health or perhaps a body in any way. Thus, hypnotherapy is going to make you understand you're not punishing yourself by abstaining from these foods, but you're doing that to enhance your overall being.

Preparing for relapse Our brains have been taught to think that relapsing from a journey or perhaps goal is actually a sinful act, as it's a reason to give up. Nevertheless, hypnosis gives us the chance of relapsing differently. The relapse becomes a chance to look at what went wrong, and learn from it, then get ready for any future temptation.

Modifying Behaviors

We are able to only achieve great goals by taking small steps at a time. Hypnosis empowers us to take the step for these little changes, which eventually end up in bigger goals. For example, when you consistently reward yourself with high-calorie content and sugary foods, you'll, over time, select a healthier reward through hypnosis.

Visualizing Success

Hypnosis is a great motivator. It enables us to see results and explore how that impacts the emotional feelings of ours. You may be in a position to visualize your future self telling others how easy it's to lose some weight.

Getting Started with Rapid Weight Loss Hypnosis Do you wish to begin your weight loss journey now? To begin, you have a number of different options. One of the options would be to visit a certified hypnotherapist who'll offer you face-to-face hypnosis sessions.

Conversely, you might schedule a session with a hypnotherapist via a virtual conference. Additionally, you may consider recorded hypnosis for self-training. The three common hypnosis options include:

One-on-one hypnosis sessions - This session allows you to identify the unconscious mental barriers that may prevent you from achieving the goal of yours. When you acknowledge the barriers of yours, you are going to be in a position to think of useful strategies to get over them.

Below are actually the things that happen during one-on-one hypnosis for weight loss:

The hypnotherapist is going to guide you into reaching the state of deep relaxation or perhaps hypnosis

When you feel completely relaxed, the therapist is going to be in a place to access the subconscious mind of yours, such as the survival mechanisms of yours and innate instincts.

The hypnotherapist will then use soothing worded scripts to explore the reasons of yours for overeating and later suggest brand new strategies of thinking through the use of visualization. The process allows you to manage any of the therapist's suggestions that you're no happy with.

Guided hypnosis sessions - This hypnosis technique entails hypnosis sessions that give you the advantage of mobility. You are going to be in a position to start the sessions when you're ready and can just make use of them when you're on vacation and even at home. The recorded sessions are able to get you through the process of weight loss, including suggestions that are actually valuable to you.

Self-conducted hypnosis sessions - A benefit of this alternative is the point that it's free of charge. With this situation, you are going to take up the job of the hypnotherapist by use of a memorized script to be able to induce hypnosis and in the end deliver positive suggestions. The primary drawback of the strategy is the fact that it may be confusing at times since you might not be aware of what you're doing in the process; thus, you might not have the ability to meet the weight loss goals of yours.

What to Expect in a Hypnotherapy Session?

Hypnotherapy sessions are able to vary in methodology and length, depending on the professional. Nevertheless, on average, a session takes lasts for forty-five minutes to sixty minutes but may go for as long as three to four hours for weight loss patients. The basic procedure entails lying down, relaxing with eyes closed, and letting the therapist guide you through suggestions, which will help you achieve the goals of yours.

Through the story of the weight loss journey of yours, a hypnotherapist has the ability to train your mind towards what's food that is healthy and away from food items that are unhealthy. Even though you are going to be in an unconscious state of mind, the procedure doesn't make you do what you're unwilling to. Someone in a hypnotic trance will literally be between being asleep and wide awake. Therefore, you're completely aware of the recommendations made by the hypnotherapist, and as such can control or perhaps possibly stop the progression.

The amount of sessions required in total per person also differs based on your own response to the quick weight loss hypnosis. Some would take as little as 3 to 4 weeks, while others might need up to eight to fifteen sessions.

REPEAT WORDS AND THOUGHTS

Experts estimate that an average adult experiences sixty thousand thoughts in a day. Fifty thousand of these are harmful. A whopping eighty percent of our thoughts are negative and unproductive. Repetitive negative thoughts can cause illness and negative outcomes in our lives. Words have a remarkable effect on our lives. They provide us with a means to share our selves and our life experiences with others. The words we regularly use affect the experiences we have in our lives. By switching up your vocabulary, you can switch up your life.

Repetition is a powerful learning tool, as it is known as the "mother" of all learning. Hypnotherapists utilize repetition wisely to pack on all aspects of hypnosis. That is the same reason that relaxes the mind during repetitive hypnosis. It is said that if something frequently happens to a desired degree or amount, you will be persuaded. That is why adverts will play consistently and on repeat because repetition is about creating a familiar pattern in abundance. When you experience something over and over again, the mind understands the phenomena causing the experience to become lodged in your memory. It is repeated so many times that it becomes convincing and, to some extent, nagging. Like when a chewing gum song will not leave your mind, and you keep repeating it all day long.

35

Repetitive thought has made its way into our lives through many channels. Remember the Lord's Prayer? We can recite it by heart because it was pounded in us at an early age. So were nursery rhymes like "Row your boat." Repetition is present in songs, musical notes, prayers, chants, mantras, and many other forms of literary works. We assign weight and importance to our thoughts to determine which ones stay longer in our minds. Repetition is often reacted to as a social cue from a colleague. When people witness something done repetitively, they too begin to do it. That is how social media has become the plague it is.

When emotions are linked to certain things, repetition can be used as a trigger to awaken those emotions. The hypnotic triple is a hypnosis rule of thumb in some schools that states that something is suggested three times to culminate an effect. Not merely saying the words thrice, but also including the theme and any emotion that may be associated with it. The mind enjoys repetition because it is calming, and calming is always good. Therefore, reconstructing your subconscious mind to have dominant positive beliefs, thoughts, and habits, the more favorable your outlook on life will be.

Repetition and the Subconscious Mind

Your subconscious mind is impartial, unrelenting, and faithful. It does most of the sifting through all of our thoughts and relates them with our senses then communicates with the conscious mind through emotions. The subconscious mind collects your thoughts and stimuli from your environment and works on forming reactions to it. For example, you may see a particular person, perhaps your neighbor and feel dislike; you may even form a scowl. Yet, you have never exchanged three words with your neighbor. Why do you feel like this towards him/her? The information you fed your subconscious.

The illusory truth effect is a phenomenon where something arbitrary becomes true because it was repeated over and over again when no one was paying any attention to it.

However, we do not know what the unconscious mind is working on because it does its works "behind the scenes." We cannot "sense" is hard at work, nor can we stop its processes. The good news then is that you can feed your mind with certain notions and ideals to elicit the emotions you have associated with them. Do not think, however, that the subconscious mind listens to reason; remember, it remains an impartial participant in your everyday life. Take an example and remember when you tried to reason with an irrational phobia- of heights or tight spaces- for example. The conscious mind knows for a fact that there is nothing to fear, but you cannot help reacting in a particular way to these fears like getting sick, for example, and feeling dizzy.

Therefore, because your subconscious mind goes in the direction you command it if you repeatedly affirm positive thoughts such as "I am beautiful," or "I can do this," you will automatically begin to develop a different attitude towards yourself. You will develop an inner outlook of your life which will gingerly propel you toward recognizing and taking advantage of the opportunities that come knocking at your door. The conscious mind can willingly train the subconscious mind and test the outcome using your life experiences. An excellent example of this is the power of autosuggestion. Have you heard of a vision board? They are ideas or fantasies that you pin up on a board that is strategically placed near the eye line. The more you repeatedly see the board, the more information you are giving the subconscious mind. After a while, check to see if there are any notable improvements in your life.. For most people, it takes roughly three months to see some progress, depending on how powerful your autosuggestions are.

Affirmations and Belief

Beliefs are formed by repetitive thought that has been nourished over and over for an extended period. Affirmations are positively charged proclamations or pronouncements repeated several through the day, every day. These words are often terse, straightforward, memorable, and repetitive. Affirmations are phrased in the present tense, and they lead to belief. The most crucial element of any self-improvement process is to set an intention. Muhammud Ali once said that "It is the repetition of affirmations that cause belief, and when the beliefs become deep convictions, that is when things start to happen."

Let's say you intend to shed some weight. That being the sole goal, it is paramount that all your efforts are focused on achieving it. Therefore, affirmative statements should be in the lines of, "Shedding pounds is as easy as packing them on," "I am what I eat," "A healthy mind is a healthy body," "I feel beautiful on the outside as I do on the inside," and so on. Keep in mind that not all the words you utter will yield results. For affirmations to work, they have to be coupled with visualization and a feeling of conviction.

Therefore, it is advisable to focus more on positive thoughts than negative thoughts and for a prolonged period.

Remember to use words that resonate with you. The affirmations need not be empty for you. They ought to have a close relation and meaning attached to them. The proper statements for the appropriate situation goes a long way in achieving success.

You can try repeating your affirmations before you go to bed. As the brain gets ready to go on "autopilot" mode, the subconscious mind becomes more active, thereby absorbing the last bits of information for the day. Repeating affirmations before you sleep not only makes you slip into dreamland in a more confident and relaxed state but also helps to convince the mind.

You might begin to wonder why, if affirmations work, they are not used to get out of "tricky" situations. For example, if you are feeling sick, would you proceed to state, "I am cured. Am I well"? Affirmations work best with an aligned state of mind. If you believe to be well, it is more likely that you will begin to notice a decline in symptoms. If you do not believe in your affirmations, you will continue to battle through the temperature and other physical discomforts.

Finding the right words to use can be a stroll in the park; however, remembering to repeat these words, severally could present itself as a challenge. The other obstacle you might face is having two conflicting thoughts. One of them is the carefully considered affirmation, while the other is a counterproductive negation. Try the best you can to disprove the negative thoughts but do not feed them time nor energy. It will be quite challenging to believe affirmations too at the beginning. However, as time goes on, it will become easier to convince yourself. Practice makes perfect.

Affirmations seem to work because:

- The act of repeating positive statements anchors your thoughts and energy, driving you toward their fulfillment

- Affirmations program the subconscious mind, which in turn processes your reactions to circumstances.

- The more frequently you repeat the affirmations, you become more attuned with your environment. You start seeing new opportunities, and your mind opens up to new ways of fulfilling your goals.

Repetition and Hypnosis

Hypnosis aims at the subconscious part of our minds to elicit lasting behavioral changes. As we have already established, repetition relaxes the mind, and when it is employed in hypnosis, the patient arrives at a state of extreme relaxation. Hypnotic suggestions can yield positive outcomes provided the intentions are set. There are two techniques used to harness the power of repetition in hypnosis.

Listen then Repeat

To bring about success during hypnosis, you must be a good listener. When someone is speaking to you, listen cautiously to both their verbal and non- verbal cues. See what both their conscious and subconscious minds are telling you. If possible, note them down.

Then say it back to them. Repeat their suggestions back to them in the language they used. When you say something in a similar tone and style, the person tends to take it as "The Gospel." Notwithstanding, they feel heard and find their thoughts acceptable when they are repeated. For example, if someone says to you "I want to shed some weight to feel more like myself," you may report back to them, "You have shed some weight, and you are feeling more like yourself." Suppose you said, "You are thin, and you are feeling more like yourself." That suggestion would be utterly useless because the language used was different, therefore ineffective.

Repetitive Themes

Because themes can mean different things to different people, they become a powerful suggestive tool. Let's say a specific client always talks about one particular direction in all the meetings. Losing weight and becoming more of themselves, for instance. Take the recurrent theme and run with it. The best hypnotherapists deliver the same piece of information is a variety of ways through repetition to reinforce the principle.

You can use repetitive themes to formulate smart suggestions that are more powerful. If the subject is narrow and too specific, allow your client to broaden the topic and use the information to generalize their theme.

When appropriately applied, both techniques offer simplicity and effectiveness because hypnotherapy patients have the solutions within themselves, not to mention the brain is soothed by repetition. Therefore, the power of personal suggestion is comfortable and safe.

Using Affirmations During Self-hypnosis

It is important to reiterate that set and setting are of paramount concern. That means that it is advisable to conduct self-hypnosis in an environment where you are not likely to be disturbed- not while operating machinery or working. Let the people in your proximity know that you will be taking a nap (because hypnosis is much like falling asleep- except with heightened sensitivity) this way; you will not be interrupted.

Step 1: Write Your Script

Ensure that the text includes the beginning that is the relaxation technique. Here, you will add the repetitive sounds and, if possible, visions of the ocean, if you love the ocean waves, or the sound of falling rain, or perhaps the forest. This element will relax you, and you will begin to feel physically relaxed and comfortable.

While you are in the relaxed space, repeat your affirmations about ten to fifteen times with natural deep breaths between each mantra. Continue enjoying the comfortable space you are in, taking in the smells, sights, sounds, and temperature. As you draw in all the senses from the space you are in, add to them the emotions triggered that particular "safe" space. As you start to feel, repeat the affirmations one more time. The conclusion of

44

your script should include a dissociation between the trance state and the reality.

Step 2: Record Your Script

Talk slowly into the recording device. Slow your pace and remember your intention for doing this. The result will be more impactful if you slow your roll and allow the subconscious mind to absorb the words as you say them. The affirmations should include statements like, "I am 10-pounds lighter," "I have control over my body," and the like.

Step 3: Find a Quiet, Comfortable Space Where You Will Remain Uninterrupted for a Few Minutes

Keep in mind that when you are attempting a hypnotherapy session, the body temperature tends to fall below average. You can prepare for this using blankets or warm clothing. Put on your earpieces and listen to your recording. Become aware of your eyelids getting heavier and heavier as you gradually close your eyes. Remember to maintain a steady breathing motion-not too fast, not too slow. The breaths should be natural, do not struggle or pant for air. With every breath, feel yourself becoming more relaxed.

All the while, keep your mind's eye focused on the repetitive swing of the pendulum. Count slowly downwards. Start from a comfortable number, perhaps eight or ten, and with each number take a deep breath into relaxation. Believe that when you finish the countdown, you will have arrived at your ideal trance state. Once you arrive, it is time to pay attention to your affirmations.

Step 4: Listen to Recording Every Day

Commitment is key. As you listen to your affirmations, make sure to repeat them.

It is also necessary to clear your mind before attempting to get into a hypnotic state. There are several ways of clearing the mind; for example, in the advent of hypnosis, a pendulum was used to draw the attention of the mind and maintain it. The repetitive motion of the swing causes the mind to slip into a trance state. The more you repeat the process of self-hypnosis, the easier it will become for you to reach a hypnotic state, and successfully alter your life.

The law of repetition states that repetition of behavior causes it to be more potent as each suggestion acted upon creates less opposition for the following suggestions. If you are looking to change your habits, it is of uttermost importance that you are prepared to put in the work. Reprogramming the mind towards

46

more real life-fulfilling goals can be an uphill climb because when habits form, they become harder to break and more comfortable to follow for all organs involved. However, all of that is learned in muscle memory. That is why repetition is emphasized. Meaning that because the mind is a muscle, it can be trained to take in more information or rewrite existing knowledge. Just like the gym, it requires a commitment to see the results. As you practice repetition frequently, maintain actionable momentum on the subconscious and conscious levels of learning. Repetition is how successes are created.

STOP EMOTIONAL EATING WITH HABITS AND AFFIRMATIONS

What Is Emotional Eating?

People usually eat to beat physical hunger. However, some people are relying on food as a source of comfort or addressing their negative emotions. Some also use food as a reward whenever they achieve their goals or when celebrating special events like birthdays or weddings.

When you use food as a cover or a solution for extreme emotions, then you suffer from emotional eating. The feelings that trigger your eating are mostly negative, for example, stress, loneliness, sadness, or when you are grieving. However, it is not only the negative emotions that can cause emotional eating; some positive emotions such as happiness or feelings of comfort can also trigger emotional eating.

There's a difference in the way folks use food to address the emotions theirs. Although some folks depend on food when they're in the middle of the life situations of theirs, others may find comfort in food shortly after the situation is actually over. They use food as a healing tool.

The explanation for emotional eating is that people use food to provide a distraction from the real problems they are facing.

Food can also be used to enhance the emotions you are going through. The feelings you get from eating then create a habit where you utilize food every time you are faced with similar situations.

A problem associated with emotional eating is that it may prevent you from utilizing other adaptive approaches to problems. You should also know that emotional eating doesn't solve the issues you are going through. If anything, it only serves to make you feel worse. After eating, the original emotional problem remains unsolved, and on top of it, you find yourself feeling guilty of overeating. It's, therefore, crucial for you to recognize the issue of emotional eating as well as to take timely, appropriate measures to stop it.

How to Recognize Emotional Eating

The absolute best way to discover in case you are suffering from emotional eating will be to find out whether you always eat since you are hungry or perhaps you eat impulsively. It is best to focus on the feelings of yours and just how you usually cope with them. Find out in case you're utilizing food just for hunger, or perhaps you're unconsciously overeating.

Once you are sure you have an emotional eating problem, take appropriate steps to stop it. This is because not all the food you eat is healthy. You will once in a while, find yourself eating unhealthy food such as junk food and sweets, which could be detrimental to your health.

Common Features of Emotional Hunger

It is easy for you to mistake emotional hunger for normal physical hunger. You, therefore, need to learn how to make a distinction between the two forms of hunger. The following are some of the hints you can use to tell the difference between the two kinds of hunger:

Emotional Hunger Comes Unexpectedly

You tend to experience emotional hunger suddenly. The feelings of craving will then overwhelm you, forcing you to look for food urgently. On the other hand, feelings of physical hunger tend to grow gradually. Also, when you are physically hungry, you will not be overwhelmed suddenly by hunger, not unless you have gone for days without food.

Emotional Hunger Desires for Some Specific Food

If you are physically hungry, any food is right for you. Physical hunger is not too selective on the type of food to consume. You will feel satisfied eating healthy food like fruits and vegetables. On the other hand, emotional hunger has a tendency to be selective on the food to ingest. Typically, emotional hunger craves unhealthy foods like junk food, snacks, and sweets. The craving for these foods tends to be overwhelming and urgent. You may experience strong desires for such food as pizza or cheesecake, and you have no appetite for any other type of food.

Emotional Eating Lacks Concern for Consequences

If you are involved in emotional eating, then in most cases, you find yourself eating without any concern about the consequences of overeating on your general wellbeing. You also eat without paying attention to the food you are consuming. You are not concern about the quality of the food or their nutritional value. All that you care about is actually the amount of food to satisfy your craving. The objective of yours is going to be to eat as much food as you can.

On the other hand, when you're consuming due to physical hunger, you are going to be mindful of the amount and also the quality of food you're consuming. You will be concern about the health benefits of the food you are eating. You will also choose to eat a very well-balanced diet, which will prevent your body from overeating junk foods.

Emotional Hunger Is Insatiable

If you are suffering from emotional eating, your hunger cannot be satisfied no matter the amount of food you have consumed. Hunger, like a craving, will refuse to get out of your mind. You are going to keep craving for increasingly more food, and soon, you'll find yourself eating continuously without a pause.

On the other hand, physical hunger is satisfied the moment your stomach is full. You may experience feelings of physical hunger only during specific times of the day. This could be the response of your body once you have conditioned it to receive food at particular times of the day.

Emotional Hunger Is Located on Your Mind

Unlike physical hunger, the craving for food originates from your mind.

Emotional hunger involves the obsession originating from your mind on some specific type of food. You find yourself unable to ignore or overcome this obsession. You then give in to it and reach for your favorite food.

On the other hand, physical hunger originates from the stomach. You feel the hunger pang from your stomach. You can also occasionally feel growling from your belly whenever you are hungry.

Emotional Hunger Comes with Guilt and Regrets

When you are suffering from emotional eating, deep down, you know your eating doesn't come with any nutritional benefits. You will then have feelings of guilt or even shame. You know you are doing your health a lot of harm, and you may start regretting your actions. On the other hand, physical eating involves eating to satisfy your hunger. You won't suffer any feelings of shame or guilt for meeting your bodily needs.

Causes of Your Emotional Eating

For you to succeed in putting a stop to your emotional eating habits, you need to find out what triggers them. Find out the exact situations, feelings, or places that make you feel like eating whenever you are exposed to. Below are some of the common causes of emotional eating:

Stress

One symptom of stress is hunger. You tend to experience the feeling of hunger whenever you are stressed. When you are stressed, your body responds by producing a stress hormone known as Cortisol. When this hormone is produced in high quantities, it will trigger a craving for foods that are salty or sugary in nature as well as any fried food. These are the food which gives you a lot of instant energy and pleasure.

If you don't control stress in your life, you will always be seeking relief in unhealthy food.

Boredom

You could be eating to relieve yourself of boredom. You can also resort to eating to beat idleness. Besides, you may be using food to occupy your time because you don't have much to do. Food can also fill your void and momentarily distract you from the hidden feelings of directionless and dissatisfaction with yourself. Whenever you feel purposeless, you tend to reach out for food to make you feel better. However, the truth is that food can never be a solution to any of your negative emotions.

Childhood Habits

Emotional eating could be a result of your childhood habits. For example, if your parents used to reward your good behaviors with foods such as sweets, ice cream, or pizza, you may have carried these habits to your adulthood.

You will find yourself rewarding yourself with your childhood snack whenever you accomplish a given task. You can also be unconsciously eating because of the nostalgic feelings of your childhood. This happens when you always cherish the delicacies you used to eat in your childhood. Food can also serve as a powerful reminder of your most cherished childhood memories, for example, if you were eating cookies with your dad during your outings together. Whenever you miss your dad, your first instinct is to reach out for the cookies.

Social Influences

Sometimes, you might have to go out with friends of yours and also have a great time. During such outings, you can share a meal to relieve stress. However, such social events can lead to overeating. You can find yourself overeating at the nudge of your close friends or family, who encourages you to go for an extra serving. It is easy to fall into their temptation.

Avoiding Emotions

You may use eating as a way of temporarily avoiding the emotions you are feeling, such as the feeling of anxiety, shame, resentment, or anger. Eating is a perfect way to prevent negative distractions, albeit temporarily.

Habits and Practices, You Can Use to Overcome Emotional Eating to Lose Weight

Practice Healthy Lifestyle Habits

You will handle life's shortcomings better when you are physically strong, happy, and well-rested. However, if you are exhausted, any stressful situation you encounter will trigger the craving for food. In this regard, you need to make physical exercise part of your daily routine. You also need to have enough time to sleep to feel rested. Moreover, engage yourself in social activities with others. Create time for outings with family or close friends.

Practice Mindfulness by Eating Slowly

When you eat to satisfy your feelings rather than your stomach, you tend to eat so fast and mindlessly that you fail to savor the taste or texture of your food. However, when you slow down and take a moment to savor every bite, you will be less likely to indulge in overeating. Slowing down also helps you to enjoy your food better.

Slowing down when eating is a vital part of mindful eating. It will also help you to get full in a short time. Learn to take a few minutes to consider the texture, smell, and shape of the food you are eating.

Accept All Your Feelings

Emotional eating is often triggered by feelings of helplessness over your emotions. You lack the courage to handle your feelings head-on, so you seek refuge in food. Nevertheless, you have to be aware of the feelings of yours. Learn to overcome the emotions of yours by accepting them. When you do this, you regain the courage to deal with some feelings that trigger your emotional eating.

Take a Moment Before Giving in to Your Cravings

Typically, emotional eating is sudden and mindless. It takes you by surprise, and often you may feel powerless in stopping the urge to eat. However, you can control the sudden urges to reach for food if you take a brief moment of 5 minutes before you give in. This allows you a brief moment to reconsider your decisions and eventually get the craving out of your mind.

Find Other Alternative Solutions to Your Emotion

Actively look for other solutions to address your emotional feelings other than eating. For instance, each time you feel lonely, rather than eating, reach out for the phone of yours and call that person that usually puts a smile on the face of yours. Look for good alternatives to food that you can rely on to feel emotionally fulfilled. If you feel anxious, learn to do exercises.

Know Your Weakness

You also need to know the specific type of food you have a problem limiting. For example, if you usually have a rough time controlling the number of fries you eat before going to bed, then you need to keep the fries out of your house. Instead, eat healthier food like apples, peanut butter, and veggies before you go to bed.

Don't Avoid Eating All Your Favorite Food

If you practice strict eating patterns, you will be forced to get rid of all your favorite food. While this seems a logical step to stop overeating, it often is counterproductive. It will eventually make you feel deprived, and you may resort to binge eating on the forbidden food. Instead, choose to eat whole, unprocessed food and make room for occasional favorite food like fries, candy, chocolate, and pizza.

Affirmations

Affirmations are an excellent tool to use alongside hypnosis to help you rewire your brain and improve your weight loss abilities. Affirmations are necessarily a tool that you use to remind you of your chosen "rewiring" and to encourage your brain to opt for your newer, healthier mindset over your old unhealthy one. Using affirmations is an important part of anchoring your hypnosis efforts into your daily life, so you must use them on a routine basis.

When using affirmations, you must use relevant ones that are going to support you in anchoring your chosen reality into your present reality. In this chapter, we will explore exactly what affirmations are and how they work, how to pick ones that are going to work for you, and 300 affirmations that will help set you on your way.

What Are Affirmations, and How Do They Work?

Anytime you repeat something to yourself out loud, or in your thoughts, you affirm something to yourself. We use affirmations consistently, whether we consciously realize it or not. For example, if you are on your weight loss journey and repeat "I am never going to lose the weight" regularly, you are affirming that you are never going to succeed with weight loss. Likewise, if you are consistently saying, "I will always be fat" or "I am never going to reach my goals, you are affirming those things to yourself, too.

When we use affirmations unintentionally, we often find ourselves using affirmations that can be hurtful and harmful to our psyche and our reality. You might find yourself locking into becoming a mental bully toward yourself as you consistently repeat things to yourself that are unkind and even downright mean. As you do this, you affirm a lower sense of self-confidence, a lack of motivation, and a commitment to a body shape and wellness journey that you do not want to maintain.

Affirmations, whether positive or negative, conscious, or unconscious, are always creating or reinforcing the function of your brain and mindset. Each time you repeat something to yourself, your subconscious mind hears it and strives to make it a part of your reality. This is because your subconscious mind is responsible for creating your reality and your sense of identity. It creates both around your affirmations since these are what you perceive as being your absolute truth; therefore, they create a "concrete" foundation for your reality and identity to rest on. If you want to change these two aspects of yourself and your experience, you will need to change what you are routinely repeating to yourself so that you are no longer creating a reality and identity rooted in negativity.

To change your subconscious experience, you need to consciously choose positive affirmations and repeat them constantly to help you achieve the reality and identity that you truly want. This way, you are more likely to create an experience reflecting what you are looking for, rather than an experience that reflects what your conscious and subconscious mind has automatically picked up on.

The key with affirmations is that you need to understand that your brain does not care if you create them on purpose. It also does not care if you are creating healthy and positive ones or unhealthy and negative ones.

All your subconscious mind cares about is what is repeated to it, and what you perceive as your absolute truth. It is up to you and your conscious mind to recognize that negative and unhealthy affirmations will hold you back, prevent you from experiencing positive experiences in life, and result in you feeling incapable and unmotivated. Alternatively, consciously choosing healthy and positive affirmations will help you create a healthier mindset and an identity that serves your well-being on a mental, physical, emotional, and spiritual level. From there, your responsibility is to consistently repeat these affirmations to yourself until you believe them, and you begin to see them being reflected in your reality.

How Do I Pick and Use Affirmations for Weight Loss?

Choosing affirmations for your weight loss journey requires you first to understand what you are looking for, and what types of positive thoughts are going to help you get there. You can start by identifying your dream, what you want your ideal body to look and feel like, and how you want to feel as you achieve your dream of losing weight. Once you have identified your dream, you need to identify what current beliefs you have around the dream that you are aspiring to achieve. For example, if you want to lose 25 pounds so that you can have a healthier weight, but you believe that it will be incredibly hard to lose that weight, then you know that your current beliefs are that losing weight is hard. You need to identify every single belief surrounding your weight loss goals and recognize which ones are negative or are limiting and preventing you from achieving your goal of losing weight.

After you have identified which of your beliefs are negative and unhelpful, you can choose affirmations that will help you change your beliefs. Typically, you want to choose an affirmation that will help you completely change that belief in the opposite direction. For example, if you think "losing weight is hard," your new affirmation could be "I lose the weight effortlessly." Even if you do not believe this new affirmation right now, the goal is to repeat it to yourself enough that it becomes a part of your identity and, inevitably, your reality. This way, you are anchoring in your hypnosis sessions, and you are effectively rewiring your brain in between sessions, too.

As you use affirmations to help you achieve weight loss, I encourage you to do so in a way that is intuitive to your experience. There is no right or wrong way to approach affirmations, as long as you use them regularly. Once you feel yourself effortlessly believing in an affirmation, you can start incorporating new affirmations into your routine to continue to use your affirmations to improve your overall wellbeing. Ideally, you should always be using positive affirmations even after seeing the changes you desire, as affirmations are a wonderful way to help naturally maintain your mental, emotional, and physical well-being.

What Should I Do with My Affirmations?

After you have chosen what affirmations you want to use, and which ones are going to feel best for you, you need to know what to do with them! The simplest way to use your affirmations is to pick 1-2 affirmations and repeat them to yourself regularly. You can repeat them anytime you feel the need to re-affirm something to yourself or repeat them continually even if they do not seem entirely relevant. The key is to make sure that you are always repeating them to yourself so that you are more likely to succeed in rewiring your brain and achieving the new, healthier, and more effective beliefs that you need to improve the quality of your life.

In addition to repeating your affirmations to yourself, you can also use them in many other ways. One way that people like using affirmations is by writing them down. You can write your affirmations down on little notes and leave them around your house, or you can make a ritual out of writing your affirmations down a certain amount of times per day in a journal so that you can routinely work them into your day. Some people will also meditate on their affirmations, meaning that they essentially meditate and then repeat the affirmations to themselves repeatedly in a meditative state. If repeating your affirmation to yourself like a mantra is too challenging, you can also say your chosen affirmations to yourself on a voice recording track and then repeat them on a loop while you meditate. Other people will create recordings of themselves repeating several affirmations into their voice recorder and then listening to them on loop. At the same time, they work out, eat, drive to work, or otherwise engage in an activity where affirmations might be useful.

If you want to make your affirmations effective and get the most out of them, you need to find a way to essentially bombard your brain with this new information. The more effectively you can do this, the more your subconscious brain will pick up on it and continue to reinforce your new neural pathways with these new affirmations. Through that, you will find yourself effortlessly and naturally believing in the new affirmations that you have chosen for yourself.

How Are Affirmations Going to Help Me Lose Weight?

Affirmations are going to help you lose weight in a few different ways. First and foremost, and probably most obvious, is the fact that affirmations are going to help you get in the mindset of weight loss. To put it simply: you cannot sit around believing nothing is going to work and expect things to work for you. You need to be able to cultivate a motivated mindset that allows you to create success. If you're not able to think that it is going to come true: trust that it won't come true.

As your mindset improves, your subconscious mind will start changing other things within your body. For example, rather than creating desires and cravings for things that are not healthy for you, your body will begin to create desires and cravings for things that are healthy for you. It will also stop creating inner conflict around making the right choices and taking care of yourself. You may even find yourself falling in love with your new diet and your new exercise routine. You will also likely find yourself naturally leaning toward behaviors and habits that are healthier for you without having to try so hard to create those habits. In many cases, you might create habits that are healthy for you without even realizing that you are creating those habits. Rather than having to consciously become aware of the need for habits, and then putting in the work to create them, your body and mind will naturally begin to recognize the need for better habits and will create those habits naturally as well.

Some studies have also suggested that using affirmations will help your brain and subconscious mind govern your body differently. For example, you may be able to improve your body's ability to naturally digest things and manage your weight by using affirmations and hypnosis. In doing so, you might be able to subconsciously adjust which enzymes, chemicals, and hormones are actually created within your body to help with things like digestive functions, energy creation, and other weight and health related concerns that you might have.

In the next half of this chapter, we will explore more than 300 affirmations you can rely on to help you lose your weight, increase your health, and feel better overall. You can use these affirmations as they are, or you can adjust them to match what you need for your belief system. If you do rewrite them, make sure that you create ones that directly reflect what you need to hear so that you can change your beliefs to those that are more supportive and less limiting.

Affirmations for Beauty

When we're in the process of changing the way our bodies look, it could be challenging to remember you're beautiful at all stages of the journey of yours, including the parts you do not like. Having affirmations to help you affirm your beauty to yourself will increase your self-esteem, self-confidence, and self-worth while also helping you generally feel better about yourself. Plus, the more beautiful you feel, the more likely you are to invest in your physical wellness and appearance, meaning that you will become even more motivated to nourish yourself well and exercise properly so that you can lose weight for good.

I am beautiful inside and out.

The happier I feel, the more beautiful I become.

When I am happy with myself, I am beautiful.

My skin is clear, healthy, and glowing.

My body is beautiful.

I have clean, smooth, and soft skin.

I love admiring myself in the mirror.

I am a beautiful person.

I am grateful for my beautiful body.

Each day, my body becomes more beautiful.

I am blessed with natural beauty.

My body is sexy.

I have a healthy, attractive body.

Being beautiful comes naturally for me.

My body is naturally beautiful.

My body shape is flattering.

My unique appearance is so beautiful.

I have a great sense of style.

I present myself with confidence and grace.

I am full of health.

I am a youthful person.

I am comfortable in my own skin.

I enjoy being admired by myself and others.

I am beautiful as I am.

My mind, body, and spirit are beautiful reflections of who I am.

I am happy with myself as I am.

I radiate true beauty.

I choose to laugh and enjoy my life because life is beautiful.

The more positive I am, the more beautiful I am.

I have beautiful features.

Even my flaws are beautiful.

My beauty radiates.

I take good care of my body and my beauty.

I am grateful for being as beautiful as I am.

My beauty shines for all to see.

I am growing more beautiful every single day.

I feel beautiful.

My features are growing more attractive every single day.

When I take care of myself, my beauty grows.

Beauty is a reflection of my inner self-love, and I love myself.

I am naturally beautiful.

My body has a naturally great shape.

The more I take care of myself, the better I look and feel.

My entire self is beautiful.

People notice how beautiful I am.

My beauty is innate.

I am uniquely beautiful.

I do not compare myself with others. I am beautiful and unique.

I see my true beauty.

I feel comfortable in my own skin.

What I see in the mirror is beautiful.

I love my entire self.

I see myself as a beautiful, loveable person.

I am beautiful.

I receive compliments with grace.

I deserve to feel beautiful.

My inner beauty shows.

I am beautiful in all ways.

I am a beautiful, radiant person.

I welcome my beauty with grace.

I choose to feel beautiful.

Affirmations for Self-Esteem

When it comes to body image, self-esteem is important. Low self-esteem can be both the cause of an undesirable body image, and the result of one. If you yourself are unhappy with how you look and feel, it could be because you lack the self-esteem to make a change, or you may feel that way because of how your health is in the present time. Either way, boosting your self-esteem now can help keep you committed to your wellness goals and can improve your ability to foster a body shape and level of health that feels more desirable for you.

I deserve a happy, healthy life and body.

I am a unique individual.

Life is fun and rewarding.

I deserve to have a body that helps me explore everything that life has to offer.

I choose to be happy and healthy right now. I love my life.

I choose to have a healthy experience.

I love and accept myself as I am.

I am successful now and forevermore.

Each day I take a step toward becoming my best self.

I deserve to love my body.

I am worthy of a positive life experience.

I inhale confidence and exhale fear.

I am passionate about myself, my life, and my wellbeing.

I am a kind and loving person.

I am full of energy and enthusiasm.

I deserve to take the best care of my body and wellbeing.

I am a flexible, adaptable individual.

I love thinking positive thoughts about myself and my body.

I surround myself with people who love me as I am.

My opinions are true to who I am.

I surround myself with people who bring out the best in me.

I choose to be my best self every single day.

I have the power to change myself for the better.

I deserve to be loved.

I deserve to feel good about myself.

I respect myself, my body, and my health deeply.

I have something special to offer.

I believe in myself.

I believe in my ability to achieve my desires.

I deserve to feel good about all of me.

Improving my self-esteem is important to me.

I can feel good about myself while working to better myself every day.

I always treat myself and my body with kindness and respect.

I am learning to love myself more and more every single day.

I choose to love myself.

I see myself with kindness.

I love myself.

I am willing to change to become the best version of me.

I approve of myself and my desires.

I care about myself, my body, and my wellness.

My commitment to myself brings me pleasure.

I praise myself freely.

I am respected by others as I am.

I rejoice in who I am.

I deserve to have a great life.

I deserve to feel good about my body.

I am worthy of wearing clothes that flatter my shape.

Each day, I am becoming more confident.

I appreciate myself.

I appreciate my body.

My body loves me.

My body deserves to feel good.

I nourish myself with healthy thoughts, food, and activities.

I care about my wellbeing.

I am willing to take better care of myself.

I treat my body with the love it deserves.

I always choose to love and care for myself.

I see my body through the eyes of love.

I see myself through the eyes of love.

I am willing to fall in love with myself.

My body is worthy of feeling it's best.

Affirmations for Self-Control

Self-control is an important discipline to have, and not having it can lead to behaviors that are known for making weight loss more challenging. If you are

struggling with self-control, the following affirmations will help you change any beliefs you have around self-control so that you can start approaching food, exercise, weight loss, and wellness in general with healthier beliefs.

I have self-control.

My willpower is my superpower.

I am in complete control of myself in this experience.

I make my own choices.

I have the power to decide.

I am dedicated to achieving my goals.

I will make the best choice for me

I succeed because I have self-control.

I am capable of working through hardships.

I am dedicated to overcoming challenges.

My mind is strong, powerful, and disciplined.

I am in control of my desires.

My mindset is one of success.

I become more disciplined every day.

Self-discipline comes easily for me.

Self-control comes easily for me.

I achieve success because I am in control.

I find it easier to succeed every day.

I see myself as a successful, self-disciplined person.

Self-control comes effortlessly for me.

Self-control is as natural as breathing.

I have control over my thoughts.

I have control over my choices.

I can trust my willpower to carry me through.

I can tap into self-control whenever I need to.

My self-control is stronger than my desire.

I am incredibly strong with self-control.

I easily maintain my self-control in all situations.

I see things through to the end.

I can depend on myself to make healthy choices.

Healthy choices are easy for me to make.

It is easy for me to control my impulses.

Self-control is my natural state.

I will keep going until I reach my goal.

I am starting to love the feeling of self-control.

I see myself as a successful person.

I have unbreakable willpower.

I have excellent self-control.

I am a highly self-disciplined person.

I succeed with every goal I create.

I am a highly intentional person.

Every day, my self-control gets stronger.

I am becoming highly disciplined.

I am successful because of my self-discipline.

I am a strong, capable person.

I am dedicated to achieving my wellness goals.

Self-control is one of my greatest strengths.

I am in complete control of this situation.

I can do this.

 I am self-aware and capable.

I can move forward with self-control and gratitude.

I always do what I say I am going to do.

I show up as my best self, and I achieve my dreams.

I have the willpower to make this happen.

I can count on myself to make the right choice.

I trust my strength to carry me through.

I am becoming stronger every day.

I make my choices with self-discipline.

I have the discipline to see this through.

I make my choices intentionally.

I am committed to my success.

Affirmations for Healthier Habits

Your habits can play a big role in your wellness. From how you eat to how you sleep and how you otherwise take care of yourself, habits are important. As you work toward losing weight and creating a healthier lifestyle, positive affirmations can help you. With the following positive affirmations, you can make committing to your healthier habits much easier.

It is easy for me to have healthier habits.

I have an easy time eating healthy food.

I eat on a regular basis.

I choose to eat healthy foods.

I move my body on a regular basis.

I foster healthy habits, so I can enjoy a healthy body.

I always choose the healthy option.

I take care of my body in the best way possible.

I am dedicated to taking care of my body.

Healthy habits come naturally to me.

I am focused on living a healthier life.

I am becoming a healthier person every single day.

I am learning to make healthier choices.

I choose to eat only healthy foods.

I am getting healthier thanks to my healthy habits.

I take the best care of my body.

Healthy habits are easy habits.

I am learning more about healthier habits every single day.

I rest when my body needs rest.

I exercise when my body needs to move.

I give my body exactly what it needs to stay healthy.

I am always learning how to have healthier habits.

I take care of my body with healthy routines.

Healthy routines make it easy for me to take care of my body.

I create healthy habits and routines that serve my unique needs.

I take care of my body the way my body needs me to.

I am willing to learn how to take care of my unique body.

I always put effort into understanding my body's needs.

I educate myself on healthy habits and enforce them as much as I can.

I am getting better at maintaining my healthy habits every single day.

I fuel my body with healthy habits.

I love engaging in healthy habits that make me feel good.

My body feels good when I live a healthy life.

Healthy habits make me happy.

I foster healthier habits in all areas of my life.

I adore having a healthier mind, body, and soul.

I live to take the best care of myself and my body.

I have an easy time fostering new habits.

My old habits shed with ease.

I pave the way for healthier habits to exist in my life.

I am committed to living a healthier, happier life.

I choose habits that help me have a higher quality of life.

My healthy habits are important to me.

I am always making healthier choices.

I find it easy to make healthy choices.

My quality of life matters, and my healthier habits help me feel better.

I love leading a healthy lifestyle.

My lifestyle is full of healthy habits.

I start my day off with a healthy morning routine.

My eating habits are healthy and nutritious.

My exercise habits are perfect for my body, my needs, and my goals.

I take care of my body in every way that I can.

I am always taking care of myself.

I have healthy boundaries that serve my healthy lifestyle.

I make healthy choices.

I always do the best that I can.

I find it easy to pick new choices.

I release habits that no longer serve me.

It is safe to try something newer and healthier.

My happiness increases tenfold when I commit to healthier habits.

My healthy habits are perfect for my needs.

Affirmations for Exercise

Exercise is necessary for healthy weight loss, but it can be challenging to commit to. Many people struggle with motivating themselves to exercise, or to exercise enough, to take proper care of their body. If you are struggling with exercising, these affirmations will help motivate you to work out or motivate you to finish your workout on a high note.

I am so excited to exercise.

I love moving my body.

I am focused and ready to exercise.

I am showing up at 100%.

Today, I will have an excellent workout.

I have the courage to see this workout through.

My body is becoming stronger every day.

I love exercising.

Exercising is fun and exciting.

I love becoming the best version of myself.

Exercising is one of my favorite activities.

Exercising makes me feel happy and healthy.

I have a strong body and mind.

I am confident about my ability to see this through.

I can feel myself becoming stronger.

I can feel myself becoming leaner.

My body is getting healthier every single day.

I am transforming my body every day.

I am creating the body I have always wanted.

Every day I am losing weight.

I am getting thinner every single day.

Each day I get closer to my ideal weight.

I am motivated to take care of my body.

I am excited to lose weight in a healthy, natural way.

My body is capable of being healthy.

I love how flexible my body is becoming.

Maintaining my ideal weight is as easy as breathing.

My weight is dropping quickly and in a healthy way.

I am dedicated to having a stronger body.

I feel myself getting stronger every single day.

My body deserves a healthy workout.

I love creating my dream body.

Having a strong body is important to me.

I am motivated to reach my fitness goals.

I am determined to have a healthier body.

I am so proud of myself for my growth.

I am strong and motivated.

I am committed to having a healthier body.

I easily become motivated to exercise.

I am capable of having a healthier body.

I feel vivacious and healthy.

I am in tune with my body.

I love how a full workout feels.

I feel all of the unhealthy toxins, leaving my body while I work out.

Every day I have more stamina.

Exercising gets easier and easier.

The more I exercise, the better I feel.

Exercising helps me sleep better.

When I look in the mirror after exercising, I love what I see.

I am strong, fit, and capable.

Every day I grow closer to my ideal body shape.

I exercise with gratitude.

I put my all into my workout sessions.

Hard work pays off.

I take a rest day when I need one.

I enjoy working out.

I love the burn that affirms my growth.

I enjoy participating in exercise.

I choose to take proper care of my body.

A healthy exercise routine and diet is all I need.

Working out helps me feel better.

I deserve to feel healthy.

While you continue to focus on your breath, I want you to keep an open mind for what is to follow. Feel your mind opening as you breathe in, allowing space for new thoughts that will nurture and support you. Allow any negative or unwanted thoughts to naturally disappear with each exhale. Continue this pattern, now.

In your open mind, repeat after me, while continuing to follow your breathing pattern:

"I am in control.

I have the power to decide.

I am in control of my desires. Self-control comes easily to me.

I can tap into self-control whenever I need to. I see things through to the end.

I love moving my body.

Today, I will have an excellent workout. I have a strong body and mind.

My body is becoming healthier every single day. I am transforming my body every day.

I am losing weight daily.

I am dedicated to taking care of my body. I choose to eat only healthy foods.

I rest when my body needs rest. I love leading a healthy lifestyle.

I am always doing the best I can. I make healthy choices.

I love myself.

I praise myself freely. I appreciate myself.

I love my body.

I am willing to change to become the best version of myself. I am a beautiful person.

I treat my body with respect it deserves. I am uniquely beautiful.

My beauty is innate.

My entire self is beautiful.

My beauty shines for all to see. I am n

aturally beautiful."

As you continue breathing, allow these words to percolate in your mind. Feel them becoming one with who you are, with your identity. Feel yourself affirming that you are a strong, capable, beautiful, worthy, and fit human being who can effortlessly lose the weight you desire to lose. Feel yourself lovingly accepting this new, healthier version of yourself. Allow yourself to become one with this new image of you. Believe the words and affirmations that you have repeated back to yourself and trust that they are true. Commit to believing them.

When you are ready, you can begin to bring your awareness back into the room around you. Allow yourself to open your eyes, return to a natural breathing rhythm, and prepare for the day ahead of you. As you do, feel yourself believing in every affirmation you heard today and trusting that it is absolutely true.

CPSIA information can be obtained
at www.ICGtesting.com
Printed in the USA
LVHW010421130121
676360LV00007B/476

9 781914 247712